The Consummate Fitness Professional

A Guide to Starting & Growing Your Personal Training Business

By Dale L. Roberts

©2015

I0421997

The Consummate Fitness Professional
A Guide to Starting & Growing Your Personal
Training Business
All rights reserved
May 18, 2015
Copyright ©2015 One Jacked Monkey, LLC
http://www.facebook.com/onejackedmonkey
ISBN-13: 978-1512275605

Table of Contents

Get a free audiobook download of *The Consummate Fitness Professional* with a 30-day trial of Audible today!

Head over to:
US Region -
https://dalelroberts.com/fitpro
UK Region -
https://dalelroberts.com/fitproUK
FR Region -
https://dalelroberts.com/fitproFR
DE Region -
https://dalelroberts.com/fitproDE

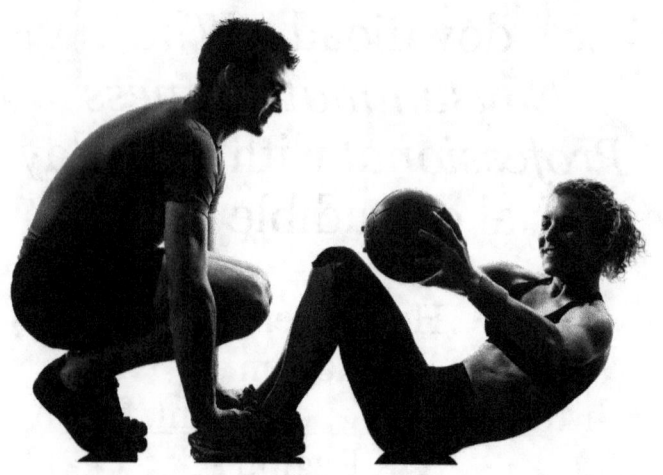

Introduction

Three years into my personal training career, a client came to me with a big smile on her face, a skip in her step, and she seemed to know something more than I did. She was diligent, stayed on track and was never wavering in pursuit of her goals. That day she hit a personal milestone and exceeded her goal of losing 30 pounds in 90 days. No doubt, it was a stellar accomplishment since it took a lot of hard work, proper eating, plenty of motivation and inspiration—most definitely a strong purpose.

We sat down afterward as I recorded her progress from her successful weigh-in. As I jotted notes, she reached into her bag and handed me a small, heavy square box. I opened it to find an etched glass trophy reading "World's Greatest Trainer: Dale 'Sweet Lou' Roberts." I teared up, unable to hide my gratitude for her kind gesture. Quickly, I wiped my eyes dry with my shirt sleeve. I composed myself and without delay, we jumped into our personal training session.

It was enough for her to spend her hard earned money on my services and her valuable time with me. Furthermore, achieving her goal was plenty of validation and reward for our work together. But, her token of appreciation was far beyond anything I'd ever expected. Her gesture left me flabbergasted and humbled.

I proudly display this trophy and keep it around to reflect on all the work I have accomplished. It is also a reminder of the work I have yet to do if I want to continue to hold the title of being the world's greatest trainer. She was one of the many people that I worked with at a small privately-owned gym. During that time, I made quite an impact on many people.

After four years with that company, I left to become an independent personal trainer. Without any coaxing, some of my diehard clients continued work with me outside the gym. I hadn't realized that I had developed a strong bond with my clientele. Upon my departure, they showed that they were invested in me, and not so much the company.

I am going to share keys to my success and further discuss concepts that are not covered in the traditional personal training certification programs or college courses. Where I have had my fair share of success, I have also seen quite a bit of failure through poor decisions. Rather than you learn the hard way as I have, I'll cover what I learned and you can build your own business quicker and stronger than I.

I'll provide some relevant answers to questions, such as:

> 1. What are some of the keys to becoming a consummate fitness professional?

2.   What are the traits to a well-rounded personal trainer?

3.   How and where do you start?

4.   Should you get a college degree or personal training certifications?

5.   Or, can you just become a personal trainer without any qualifications?

6.   How do you build your clientele?

7.   How do you maintain and grow your business simultaneously?

8.   How can you retain clients? If you cannot keep a customer, then how do you plan for that loss in revenue?

9.   How can you get referrals and create additional client leads?

I will provide you keen insights and a real world approach to your personal training business. Sure, you may know the difference between the biceps brachii and the biceps femoris. However, if you don't have a practical and logical approach to your business, then you may not have longevity in this industry. Education shows you the importance of why health and fitness. But, without knowing what your client wants, no amount of knowledge will get you far. I heard it said best—nobody cares what you know till they know that you care. *The Consummate Fitness Professional* comes in to solve the issue—to bridge the gap between education, learning and applying your craft in personal training.

Chapter 1 - Defining Your Path

It's awesome that you are considering a career as a personal trainer. As a fitness professional, you build lasting relationships, impact many lives and your efforts can echo for years after. You develop a bond with people you eventually consider friends and family. You also have the opportunity to nurture hope in people, because, in personal training, they're not necessarily just buying your services. Your clients are investing in hope. They expect to achieve something greater with you than if they were to do it alone. You play a significant role in someone's better future as a personal trainer.

There are a few things you have to consider when becoming a fitness professional. Before deciding on your education, certification, or even your liability insurance, you should think about who your ideal audience is.

I initially started personal training in 2006. Before considering a career in health and fitness, I weighed 155 pounds, had a beer belly and I really didn't care about my health. Inspired by the athleticism of sports entertainment in 1999, I quickly learned as much as I could about how to become as fit as a pro wrestling athlete. My general curiosity grew into an obsession and, before long, I was reaping the benefits from a healthy lifestyle.

Within a couple of years of eating right and exercising diligently, I built a lean 185-pound body. The results were enough for me to want to share my success with others. So, my motivation for personal training was to inspire, educate and train others to accomplish what I had. I believed my audience was going to be guys just like I was—tall and skinny with a beer belly.

In reality, my personal training career was quite the opposite from my expectations. I began working in a small, privately-owned gym as a club cleaner. I meticulously cleaned the entire gym from top to bottom, inside and out. I wanted to be the best club cleaner so that I would be noticed for my undying work ethic. Within a few days, the regional personal training manager approached me and offered me the opportunity to join the team.

Right away the company enrolled me in continuing education courses. Within four months, I received my first personal training certification with the American Council on Exercise. Soon after, I scheduled my first appointment. The day of the session, I was outwardly nervous yet happy to get my new career started. However, for my first appointment and many appointments after that, a mismatch occurred between my expectations and what happened.

My first session was with a short, middle-aged couple who couldn't even fit the exercise equipment at the gym. Also, their goals were not to put on muscle. Their goals were far from what I expected or was prepared for. They just wanted to, in their words, "Get in shape." I just assumed they would want to look and feel exactly as I did. When the workout session was over, the couple had made up their mind to do it on their own. I was crushed that I couldn't be their trainer. And worse yet, I didn't know why I never earned their interest. Analyzing the situation, I approached them in a self-serving way.

This was the wrong approach in any relationship—professional or personal. This selfish philosophy can ruin any business. I learned that what I wanted and what they wanted were not always the same. To be successful with my clients, I had to develop a plan to get them from where they were to where they wanted to go.

In fact, after that first appointment, I rarely found a scrawny guy with a beer belly, looking to put on muscle and burn off some body fat. Most clients at my gym were business people and stay-at-home moms looking to tone up and lose a few pounds. They didn't want to be muscled up and were mostly content in simply feeling better or losing ten to twenty pounds of fat.

I became frustrated and needed to change my approach and mindset for me to be successful in this business. After many setbacks, I looked for guidance from experienced trainers in our company. I became teachable and allowed the company to mold me into a better trainer. Quickly, I adapted my training style and philosophy to the demographic of the fitness club. Success seemed to come almost instantly and my schedule filled quickly.

An ideal situation for my original expectations would have been to search a gym that had the audience or demographic I was looking to work with. Sure, there were plenty of guys who were tall and skinny with a pot belly and they wanted to bulk up and cut body fat. Possibly a body builder's gym would have worked for me, but definitely not the location or the audience that I came to know.

You need to make a few choices before you become a personal trainer.
1. Why do you want to become a personal trainer?
2. What is the demographic, or segment of the population[i], you want to work with?
3. Are you willing to adapt to your audience's wants and needs?

People may spend their whole lives climbing the ladder of success only to find, once they reach the top, that the ladder is leaning against the wrong wall.
-Thomas Merton

Why Do You Want to Be a Personal Trainer?

Why do you wish to become a personal trainer? The reason I became a personal trainer was to pass on what I learned from living a healthy lifestyle. When I dropped body fat and increased muscle, I felt great, confident and better than ever. So, I wanted other people to feel the same way I did and learn from my experience.

What is your purpose or your reason for becoming a fitness professional? Your purpose is the reason why you do what you do. Think about your purpose for becoming a personal trainer. If you are getting into this business for the money, then you are going to have a lot of setbacks and heartache. You shouldn't pursue a career in the health and fitness industry for fame and fortune because these reasons will not get you much success.

This job provides you with many challenges and adversities. Clients will blame you for their setbacks and their failures. People will blow off appointments or simply stop showing up. And, competitors will undercut your services and take clientele from you. These are just a few issues that will come up in your fitness career. With a strong purpose for pursuing this career, you will overcome most problems and push past the inevitable obstacles.

Your purpose should be less about how much money you make and more about how many lives you can positively affect. When you provide consistently superior service and aim to help others, you will build a reputation, credibility, and experience. In due time, you will have a solid base of clients, a waiting list of future customers and many raving fans who spread news of your work.

"You can have everything in life you want if you will just help enough other people get what they want."

-Zig Ziglar

Eventually, you will make a substantial income, feel good about what you're doing and see many other rewards. Make no mistake, your likelihood of becoming a millionaire in this career are pretty slim. According to Salary.com, 50% of personal trainers make less than $55,344 per year and 90% of personal trainers earn less than $ 79,478 annually[ii]. Also, consider the time that some trainers work on an average day. In my experience, I knew trainers who worked upwards of 12 to 16 hours every day without a break. Yet they're not even making a six-figure salary from such long days. Additionally, these are excellent trainers who are booked full with appointments.

The good news is that I will show you how to develop a schedule that is reasonable to your lifestyle and builds a stable business. I believe that you can work smarter and not harder to make the most out of the least time.

Who is Your Audience?

The second step is for you to determine your ideal audience. Who are the people you want to work with on a regular basis? Visualize the types of clients that you feel you would best suit your interest and future skill set.

For instance:
1. Do you want to work with long-term weight loss clients?
2. Would you like to train bodybuilders or athletes?
3. Are marathon runners or triathletes?
4. What is the age group you would prefer?
5. Will your customers be children, young adults, middle-aged or senior citizens?

Knowing who your audience plays a significant role in where you work and how you train. Narrow down to what fits your interests, knowledge and skill set. It's okay if you don't have the knowledge, I'll discuss how to get the education in the next chapter. For now, at least, choose who you would like to work with on a regular basis. You aren't married to your decision and you can always change your mind later.

Once you've determined your customer avatar, find out where your audience is. This may require a little exploration in your neighborhood. Go to franchise gyms, privately-owned clubs, and personal training studios. It may help to contact mobile personal training businesses, too. If you know an experienced personal trainer, then ask them what type of clients they work with, where they're working and the kind of environment they're working in. This information gives you a better idea of where to start your personal training career.

Branding Yourself

Despite the phrase "Don't judge a book by its cover," you will be judged in all of your business. And, the first thing people judge you on is your appearance. Choosing your professional appearance and the look of your company is crucial to your success. A large part of your business is going to involve how you look, how you conduct yourself and how you want to be remembered. All of these elements are a part of your marketing and branding.

Marketing is how you advertise yourself. And, branding is how you want to be perceived within your marketing. Everyone is watching you whether you are in the gym, on the street or online (i.e. social media, websites, video).

When marketing yourself, think about how you wished to be perceived as a business and what makes the best sense to attract your ideal audience. When I worked at a privately-owned gym, I wore matching black polo shirt, dress slacks, and dress shoes. The company felt this uniform made the training staff look professional, knowledgeable and approachable. Later, when I became an independent personal trainer, I changed my work attire because I wanted to be more personal and relatable. I switched my dress code to comfortable clothing—an athletic shirt, sweat pants, and cross-training shoes. My clientele agreed that my new dress code fit my personality and training style. They didn't perceive me as the type of person wearing a polo shirt or dress slacks outside of the gym. No matter your choice in uniform, make sure it is clean, wrinkle-free and you are presentable.

Dress Professionally

At my local gym, I saw an independent personal trainer wear ripped jeans, a bedazzled ball cap, and a tank top meant for a grade school girl. In my opinion, this shows no professionalism and makes her session look more like a hangout at a bar rather than a workout in a gym.

If you are going to be a consummate pro, dress the part and make sure that you are presentable for the occasion. I recommend an athletic mesh collar shirt, comfortable pants, like sweats or pressed slacks, and a pair of comfortable tennis shoes.

Stick to conventional clothing for branding purposes. You want people to see you as an authority in your field and an established, reliable brand. Your appearance sets the standard for what people can expect when they work with you.

The reason you want to keep your attire the same is so people become programmed to seeing you and recognize you as a personal trainer. Whether it's in the gym, an apartment complex clubhouse or even in a park, people will pick you out and say, "There's that personal trainer." They are going to recognize you as a particular brand. Dressing professionally, you'll leave a real good and lasting impression. People are always watching. So remember that you should conduct and present yourself as a classy professional.

Define Your Outcome for Success

Now, set your own definition of success in business. Blindly hoping for the best is not a great business strategy. Two critical elements are:

1. What are your hours of operation
2. What kind of revenue or money do you make

Essentially, you are goal setting for your business, a similar process you use with your clients. If you don't know your target, how do you know where to aim? Pick your bullseye so that you increase the likelihood of success.

First, choose your schedule and how it fits into your life. Though I mentioned sixteen-hour days are available, this does not mean you have to commit to that type of schedule. In my personal experience, I was successful in longer days, but I became burnt out fast. I didn't have much of a personal life because I was spending all my time in the gym. Conversely, I saw better success only working six hours every weekday. Though I had a shorter schedule, I filled my day with top dollar training sessions and few breaks. This left the rest of my day free to do whatever I wanted. However long you wish to work, choose your hours of operation and adjust to what works for you.

When you have a schedule picked out, figure out what kind of income you want to earn when you're successful. If you are going to work 40 hours per week and want to make $1,000, then divide the income by the hours to figure out your hourly rate or client cost per session. Then you will know how many clients you need to have to meet your revenue goal. This sounds simple enough, but filling the hours can be daunting at first. At least, you will know what you need to do to make your business as successful as possible.

Then, figure out your long-term business goals. What kind of objectives do you have set for one year, five years and ten years? Is this the career that you'll retire from later in life? Or is this job a stepping stone to something much bigger? Think about where you are going, because much like the goals you're going to have your clients set, you need to make sure that you adhere to the same goal-setting principals for your business, too.

Lastly, what will define your success in the field of personal training? How will you know that you have made it? Before I began personal training, I envisioned what was going to be my success:

1) Validation – through testimonials, before and after photos and client endorsements

2) Busy schedule – a fully booked eight-hour day for five days per week.

3) Exceed previous annual income - Money was never a motivator, but it was a milestone indicating I grew as a professional and exceeded efforts in my previous occupations

Chapter 2 - Gaining Credibility

"Trust is built on credibility, and credibility comes from acting in others' interests before your own."

-Stephen Denny

Credibility is the quality of being believable, genuine and honest[iii]. In the health and fitness industry, if you want to be taken seriously by your peers and clientele, then you have to build credibility. And, the way to do that is to get educated, apply what you have learned and become experienced in your field.

It's important to establish yourself as a qualified fitness professional with credibility—not just as any person off the street or some random person dispensing questionable advice. You need to be credible, reliable and qualified. Additionally, you must offer sound recommendations that keep your clients safe and their workouts effective.

The personal training industry is, for the most part, unregulated, so this means that anybody can be or assume the title of a personal trainer. This should not stop you from being the best, most qualified fitness professional. Become educated and certified for the type of personal training you want to provide.

Preparing for a Career in Personal Training

There are three different ways you can prepare yourself for a career in personal training. You can take the longer route—and a worthy one—by getting a college degree. I've known many trainers that have specialized college degrees they are able to parlay into a career as a personal trainer. Then, the second route is becoming certified through a reputable fitness organization. A personal training certification verifies you know what you are doing. Lastly, the third way is doing nothing at all and simply calling yourself a personal trainer. All three routes have been used with either significant results or no success.

Getting no education or verification by an organization as being a qualified personal trainer is a poor way to establish your credibility. In a business with no regulations, there still is a liability or legal responsibility[iv] to your clientele. Since you oversee the safety of a person's well-being, you are legally responsible for instructing and fully informing your client in a proper manner. Without an endorsement from a credible source, you increase the likelihood of an unsuccessful outcome of potential litigation if a client feels you have been neglectful or improper in your training methods. This means that if you get sued, you may lose in the lawsuit without a reputable organization's endorsement.

Doctors need years of specialized training to

practice in their field. Yet you don't need to have a license, a degree, or certification to be a personal trainer. In both careers, you have a person's well-being in your hands. And, though accidents are not certain, you should decrease the likelihood by getting adequate, on-going education. In the event of an unpreventable catastrophe, you can, at least, prove your intent to do no harm to your client through evidence of being qualified through a certifying organization.

If you want to take your career seriously as a fitness professional, then you should either choose to get a college degree or a relevant certification. Once you get that college degree or certification, you will then have a particular range of education and experience that you are endorsed in and should practice within.

Scope of Practice

The range, or the extent of your knowledge application, you should work within is your scope of practice. Even though no regulations exist for personal training, why is the scope of practice so crucial?

To illustrate the point, I had a personal experience that shows what scope of practice is and how it is important from a liability standpoint. I knew a young certified personal trainer. He grew a small client base with consistent and diligent work. His real issue was that he couldn't keep clients for long because he didn't design appropriate workouts for his clients.

He would mimic an exercise video he saw, another trainer he admired or someone performing an intricate or fancy exercise.

Yet, he didn't know what the exercise did, how it was properly done or why it should be done in the first place. Sure he could guess what the movement did and bullshit his way through it. But, he didn't have a fundamental understanding or education to instruct in this exercise. Often, he would use the same workout for every client all day long, then switch the workout the next day to highlight an entirely different routine. There was no rhyme or reason to the training he provided his clients. Remember, that certain exercises may be great for one client, but not appropriate for another client. Knowing if an exercise is right for specific fitness levels and types of people is crucial in minimizing liability in your personal training business.

Widen your scope of practice by getting more education and certifications to back up your knowledge. When training, stick to what you can properly instruct and fully explain. Additionally, you should quickly determine who it is appropriate for. When you stay within your scope of practice it protects you, and most importantly, it reduces the likelihood of client risk.

The health and fitness industry can be dangerous if you aren't careful and do not choose the proper steps. Thankfully, the young man in that story never saw any injuries, but he lost a lot of clients due to his apparent lack of knowledge and training acumen. Remember, people can sense when you don't know what you're doing. This is a business where you cannot fake it till you make it. You have to stick with what you know and admit when you are in over your head.

Scope of practice comes down to education, certification and application in your skill set. If you are certified in squats, push-ups, pull-ups, and crunches, then you should stick to those exercises until you have been certified in something new. Take pride in your knowledge and be the expert in that area. When in doubt about how to handle a client, refer that person to a specialist who can properly handle their individual needs. Everyone appreciates you in the end and you gain more respect and credibility in the end.

Where to Get Your Education

Once you identify your audience, you need to get the proper training to become a fitness professional. Though a college education may take a little longer to develop the fundamentals, it is a worthy investment. With a college degree, you can widen your scope of practice and get a firm grasp on health and fitness. Consult a college counselor for advice on the right curriculum based on your goals for your personal training career. But, why should you make such a substantial investment before you know if personal training is the career for you?

I worked with personal trainers who were fresh out of college. Some floundered in their business and discovered it wasn't at all what they expected. So, before you invest in college, be sure that you attend the right institution that will not only provide an excellent education, but also, the proper tools to gain employment or to start a business. The college graduates I worked with had all of the book knowledge yet lacked fundamental skills—customer service, branding, marketing, and sales.

Before you enroll in a college program, get some experience and a better understanding of personal training. Shadow a personal trainer, hire a personal trainer or obtain a personal training certification. The first two options give you general ideas and expectations of personal training sessions. Also, it's far cheaper and requires less time to get a personal training certification as opposed to a college degree. With a personal training certification, you can start working and determine if a higher education is practical and what you expected.

When it comes to personal training certifications, there are many different options available and it's easier than ever to get one. Before you spend any money, make sure the organization has the type of personal training you want and requires continuing education to keep you up-to-date on current health and fitness information. Also, get a certification from an organization with relevant specialty certifications and advanced courses to develop your training skill set. Don't simply settle with the basic certification and strive to grow in this industry.

Additionally, some personal training schools offer a wide variety of options for your education. Before you invest in their schooling, confirm that you aren't just paying for the same personal training certification you could otherwise obtain on your own. However, if you thrive in a classroom environment and lack the discipline of getting the personal training certification on your own, then these types of schools may work for you.

Certification Cost

Most personal training certifications cost anywhere from $300 to as much as $600 to $800 dollars. Most certification programs range in price depending on a good-better-best model. All the models, or certification packages, provide the same outcome; however, you are provided more content for spending more money. Paying for the certification may get you study materials, such as, books, videos, and online courses, but it does not guarantee that you will get the certification. You must prove that you studied and retained the information by taking a test. Most credible organizations have their tests run at a proctor-run third party company. If you study hard and pass your certification test, then you become certified. The proof of certification is typically processed then mailed to you 6-8 weeks after passing the certification testing. However, the organization may provide temporary proof of certification after passing the test so that you can begin work right away. Ultimately, the investment will pay for itself if you get clients, apply what you know and continue to learn.

A little research is necessary before you spend money on a certification program. If you see a trainer who you admire or is successful in the field, then find out his certification. Next, if you plan to work for a particular employer, then find out what certifications they accept and if you need any additional credentials to possibly gain employment.

Certification Suggestions

I'll share three organizations that have been used by many successful trainers. I have no direct affiliation with these organizations nor does my opinion represent them. These are merely recommendations on what I've seen successful trainers use.

American Council on Exercise (ACE) is a widely recognized organization that certifies trainers for all types of fitness. I obtained my base certification from this organization and have used a lot of their continuing education and specialty certifications to grow my knowledge and business. They have excellent free information on their website and anybody can access it. Also, they trainer-exclusive discounts on continuing education to keep your certification updated. My experience as an ACE certified personal trainer began when I traveled to Calgary in 2006. The ACE certification was recognized and accepted by the gym owners, so I was allowed to train at their gyms. It was a relief knowing I partnered myself with a widely accepted organization.

The National Academy of Sports Medicine (NASM) has excellent, detailed material and the most thorough education I've seen for personal training. The certification process is a lot more stringent and requires more studying to pass their testing.

Lastly, the International Sports Science Association (ISSA) is another reputable organization to get your certification. They have a specialty certification called Certified Strength and Conditioning Specialists (CSCS) used by trainers who work with athletes. Much like the other two previously mentioned certification bodies, they too have continuing education, significant resources, and credibility in the health and fitness industry.

Liability Insurance

Before getting your first client, liability insurance is 100% necessary. If you are an employee at a gym, then check if they have liability insurance for their training staff. Get a copy of their liability insurance plan to file away with your personal training information. Do not go without confirming your employers have adequate liability insurance. If they do not have liability insurance, then you consider investing in your own liability insurance.

In the event your client becomes injured and sues you or your company, the liability insurance will help protect your business. Unfortunately, finding liability insurance isn't as simple as contacting your local insurance agent. Specialized insurance companies have personal training liability insurance and are experienced in guiding trainers to what fits their business needs. Most certifying organizations can refer you to the best companies and plans that cover a range of cases. Basic coverage can cost about $170 dollars or more per year and may include $1-$2 million dollars in litigation.

Can you go without liability insurance? Absolutely. Should you? No, you shouldn't go without at least the minimum liability insurance. Much like any other insurance, you get it in case of disaster. Having the right certification and liability insurance goes hand-in-hand. See your certifying organization to be referred to a good insurance company.

Necessary Tools as a Trainer

If you are an employee at a gym, most tools—a scale, body fat monitor, tape measure—may be readily available. However, if you're running a business on your own, then I highly recommend you get these tools.

You need a system for filing client information. I used an accordion file where I stored client documentation into alphabetized separators. This type of file is at any office supply store. However, technology has progressed, now a portable electronic device such as a tablet or iPad stores tons of client information. If you use any technology, then always back up your electronic information in a safe, secure place.

Each client file should have a checklist of items needed for proper and thorough documentation, including:

1) Basic client information - name, age, address, email, etc.
2) Pictures - before & after if necessary
3) Informed consent, liability waivers, permission or agreement forms
4) Goal sheets
5) Measurements
6) All workouts planned ahead and dated

Whether you use an accordion file or technology for client information, try to keep everything organized and readily available. It's a challenge to remember everyone's personal goals, specific conditions and the precautions needed for their session. When a client shows up, preparation demonstrates your dedication to quality service and responsibility. Rest assured, when you have a lot of clients coming and going, you will not regret having all of the files in order.

Organization is critical in running a successful personal training business.

Most certifications cover what tools you need according to the type of personal training you do. General tools needed in personal training are:

1) Scale
2) Tape measure
3) Digital camera
4) Body fat monitor
5) Exercise equipment required for your training session

You are responsible for having these tools ahead of any session. It doesn't look good for you if a client sees you don't have what's needed for a session. When I worked at a gym, I was horrified when I would discover that the tape measure was gone, the scale was broken or the batteries died in the body fat monitor. Having everything prepared ahead of time is crucial to your appointments. You need to appear professional and well organized; not like you are completely frazzled and surprised by missing or malfunctioning tools.

Credibility Conclusion

If you want to be taken seriously and establish a lasting business, then your credibility as a fitness professional is what determines your longevity in this business. A college degree or a certification from an accredited organization is the best way to lay a foundation for credibility in the health and fitness industry. To be the consummate fitness professional, you need to have the credentials to verify who you say you are.

Sure there are no regulations in personal training, and there may not be anybody arresting you if you train without a certification or degree. However, most liability insurance companies will not endorse you and employers are less likely to have an interest in hiring you without a qualifying certification. Getting a personal training certification may be essential if you want to succeed as a personal trainer.

Train within your scope of practice—stick to what you know and what you're certified in. Because you saw it on television or another trainer doing it, doesn't mean you should do it. If an exciting exercise interests you, then get the education and certification to train clients with it.

Protect the business you develop and grow by having not only proper education but also, minimum liability insurance. Accidents happen, even with every precaution, perfect verbal cue, and pre-planned session. And, in the rare case that someone blames you for their injury, liability insurance may protect your business, your assets and your future within the industry.

Be prepared and organized for your business. You have limited time to work with your clients, so make every second count by having all of their information filed accurately, in order and ready in advance. Any tools you need to fulfill a session should be available for all appointments. Organization and preparation will establish you as a consummate fitness professional.

Chapter 3 - Building Your Business

Business Model

After you have identified why you want to become a personal trainer and have acquired education through a certification or degree, you should develop your business plan and build your audience. After all, if you don't have a business and an audience, then you don't have a career.

First, you should know your business model or a plan for the successful operation of your business. A good business model identifies your revenue source, customer base, products, and services. The final element, financing, or how you obtain money to start and maintain your business, is crucial to the independent personal trainer/small business owner. If you work at a gym, most employers allow you to practice at their gym in exchange for a percentage of your commissions or for your compensation in hourly wages. Therefore, as an employee, financing is not an essential item to your business.

Creating a stable business model is crucial for small business owners and not as necessary for anyone seeking employment with a company. Draft out and write exactly what your business is by identifying your revenue sources, your customer base, your product, and details in financing.

Business Costs & Essentials

A good business model requires an outline of how you obtain funding or funding to get your business properly running. If you include continuing education, uniforms, tools and anything to make your business run effectively, then you should have these expenses accounted for before acquiring financing. You want to ensure your business is profitable and not creating a loss.

You can acquire some financial resources through other small business owners, area entrepreneurs, and bank loans. Asking for money to start your business requires a lot of time, research and preparation. Be sure that you have read through this whole book to get a better idea of what you need to grow a successful business. Then, find out the cost and how to categorize each item in your business. For instance, a few categories to consider are:

1) Equipment - Dumbbells, rubber bands, exercise mats, cable equipment, etc.
2) Education - continuing education to keep your practice up to current standards and renew any certifications
3) Uniform - any clothes used strictly for business purposes only
4) Travel expenses (mobile training) - gas, vehicle upkeep & maintenance, mileage reimbursement
5) Any additional items that would make your business successful

When asking for money to start your business, you must be prepared to explain a plan to pay back the loan, what is in it for loan provider, projected expenses and plan for growth and development of your business.

I would suggest bootstrapping your business, meaning you work from scratch to get your business running successfully. While it is a longer and harder road, working for an employer first is an excellent way to gradually learn and funnel money to the side so you finance your own business. Consider reserving 10% of your pay to build your independent personal training business. When you have all the money you need to begin your business, all you will have to do is put in your notice with your employers and start anew.

This method worked well for me because I used my time working with a company to save money and acquire equipment as I went along. When the time came that I felt confident to try business on my own, I took the leap of faith and found my lessons in the gym paid off.

Revenue through Training

Your clientele, or your customer base, is your primary source of income. As a business owner, you can choose to incorporate other forms of revenue, such as supplement sales, online article writing, and affiliate marketing, among others. Be sure that if you plan to sell anything outside of your normal services as a personal trainer that it stays within your scope of practice. For instance, some organizations discourage sales and endorsement of supplements due to the lack of scientific evidence and proven efficacy. If you are new to this business, keep it simple and focus on building your clientele. Develop back-end sales only when you have filled your schedule and established credibility with your audience.

Setting Your Price Point

Determine your type and value of your personal training services. Choose your session length—30 minutes, 45 minutes or 60 minutes. And, set the cost for each session length and whether you give price breaks for advance payments. Incentives to make advance purchases can benefit everyone. Good for you because you have a client for a guaranteed period of time. Great for your client because he has acquired the same services that he'd otherwise use but at a discounted price.

Also, what payment methods are you able to process and accept? Cash, credit card, and check payments are easy to handle now with various mobile applications and accessories. Regardless of the method you choose, keep accurate documentation for your accountant, your clientele, and your business records. When the option is available, always provide a receipt of payment to your clientele to avoid any issues or discrepancies.

Cost Setting for the Independent Personal Trainer

Most employers determine employee pay, whether it is salary-based or in most instances, price per trained client. Generally, employers compensate based on educational background and experience. When I worked for a company, they established the rate of a one-on-one session for a half hour at $47 and an hour session at $88. I did not have a choice on cost. If I wanted to be paid more per appointment, then I had to schedule more clients. This was the rate they chose and was part of their business model. Based on how many clients I saw on a daily basis and if I met a quota, I'd get 60% percent of the session rate. This means I received:

1) Half-hour session cost = $47, Trainer pay = $28.20
2) Hour session cost = $88, Trainer pay = $52.80

But if I saw nobody within a half hour or an hour, then I was paid nothing. Even if a client paid in advance, I wouldn't receive pay. As long as the client called off within the 24-hour window per the cancelation policy, I'd receive no money for the empty timeslot (covered further in this chapter).

As an independent personal trainer, how much are your services worth? You can decide on your own or you can do some research. Find out today's average pay and how your services figure into that standard. When I transitioned from personal training employee to self-employed trainer, I used the same cost model. But, I adjusted the cost per session at a 40% discount since I was accustomed to that pay as an employee. I was happy with the pay structure and felt I was still being paid my worth. Since my mobile training business didn't have the same amenities of the gym, I felt it was only fair to offer the rate cheaper than my former employers. This competitive price enticed more clientele to continue training for me while not undercutting my old bosses so much that it would adversely affect their bottom line.

Believing in Your Value as a Trainer

Know your value when setting your session rates as an independent trainer and stand by it. Whether you have to put it down in print—on a brochure, on a website—just stick to your worth. You represent your business and are the chief executive officer of your company. Would you allow one of your workers to downgrade or devalue one of your services?

If you determine that you are worth $50 for a half-hour session, then stay firm to $50 for a half-hour routine. You will do business with hagglers and they will try to convince you to discount your rate.

"Well, I can only afford $20 dollars per half hour" or "That's expensive!" If they don't see the value, then they're not going to afford it. If they understand the value of your service, then they will find a way to make it work. You have to know your worth, and stand by it.

Think if you put in an order at a fast food restaurant. When the price point is delivered, there is no negotiation. The only negotiation that exists is whether you will have your food or do without since you don't have the money. The same applies to your services. If you provide a stellar service, give your expertise, your time and your energy, then you should be paid accordingly.

Pricing Change

As time goes on, you may have to adjust your rates. Maybe increase or decrease it according to how the health and fitness industry is performing. Stick to a rate for a period of time and re-evaluate on a quarterly basis or every 3 months. Don't drop your prices to bring in more clientele. If you need more clients, then you need to be in front of more people. Change your marketing techniques and community outreach. The chances are likely that if you don't have many clients, then not too many people know about your business.

If you adjust your rates, be sure to track your session rates for each client, so when you bill your clients, you stay accurate with the original agreed cost. If you do an overall price increase to accommodate inflation needs for your business, then give all of your clients advance notice. You may have to express in person, by email and by letter your intent to increase rates. The most tactful way to approach a price increase is to take the time to discuss it privately with your client. Be open to client's questions and adequately prepared to address and resolve issues. People don't like paying more for the same service, but they'll be more receptive when you have a logical explanation for the increase.

When I was working for my employers, every time that I acquired a specialty certification, my rate would increase. I had to give each client an advance notice of my intent to raise the prices. Most of my clients were understanding and were fully aware that I had acquired additional education. So, they were prepared for this price increase. A few clients parted ways with me but most stayed, happy to keep my services.

Where to Work

There are two common business types in personal training—be an employee for a company and be a small business owner as an independent personal trainer. Many pros and cons exist for both types of business, so be selective about where you start and continue to work.

Working as an Employee

I highly recommend working for an employer when you first start in the business. However, choose the company wisely. You will work underneath a manager and can learn at a more deliberate pace than if you were to run your own business. You'll contribute to a team responsible for the success of the company.

The real advantage to working as an employee is you have potential clients everywhere. Assuming that the gym has plenty of member and guest traffic, you have plenty of potential clients. Be professional and provide superior service and in due time your schedule will fill up.

One disadvantage of working as an employee is competition. It's likely the company hires many excellent trainers and has only a certain number of members and guests. If there are two trainers on the personal training team and one thousand members, then there isn't much competition. But if you're in a group of twelve trainers and the gym has two hundred members, then the competition will be greater.

Hopefully, you choose a good employer with a cohesive team with a common interest in success together. After all, when you work together as a team, you are not going to filch another trainer's clients or prospects. Remember, if you work on a team, you have to see these people on a regular basis and learn to act professionally and tactfully with each other.

You will also discover other personal trainers don't always align with your health and fitness philosophies. This can work against you if you allow it. For instance, I worked with a personal trainer who gave poor service and the members complained about him. Because of his inadequate service, a lot of people had a bad view of all the personal trainers. They felt that if one personal trainer conducted himself this way, then all trainers were like him. Why would anyone want to buy from terrible trainers?

In the event you are in this type of situation, you're going to have to stand out and exceed expectations. Provide exceptional customer service or treat the customers like they want to be treated. I go out of my way to ensure clients, members, and guests feel like this is the best part of their day and it is an experience to remember. Customer service includes staying upbeat, listening to your client, responding with empathy and delivering what you say you would. And, in some cases, give a little extra something to show that you actually care about their patronage and support.

Working as an Independent Personal Trainer

The second type of personal training business is to be independent or a small business owner. As an independent personal trainer, you will have to find a place that you can call home in your personal training business. Here are a just a few examples of where an independent personal trainer can work:

1) Rent space from a gym or studio owner

2) Mobile training - travel from one location to the next; conduct your business at parks, recreation centers or homes

3) Collectively pool rent money with multiple independent personal trainers for a co-op location

Your business model should have this included in costs (i.e. rent, travel expenses). If you're an independent personal trainer, then some kind of cost is involved for you to continue to run a profitable business. I worked as a mobile personal trainer where I'd go to client homes or public parks for my appointments. Use caution on both types of locations:

1) Don't train on a floor above the ground level. This may disturb neighbors and you will have to answer to an upset

landlord or worse yet the authorities.

2) Get permission to train in all public parks. Contact the local parks and recreation to get approval. Not all parks can be used for conducting business and some require an agreement or contract signed in advance. Some parks require a percentage of revenue, too.

3) Not all clients are going to have the best environment to train in. Assess all homes before agreeing to train. Some homes are a nightmare to work in with children running amuck, spouses lounging around or a messy home filled with hazards.

Mobile business is enticing since you aren't anchored to one spot and can get a broader range of clients. Think about all the costs of a traveling business, though. Expenses can include gas money, food and miscellaneous transportation maintenance and upkeep of your vehicle. Plan out what the best fit is for you. If you limit your travel radius for clientele, then you can minimize travel costs. Though you may get a client, it wouldn't necessarily be good if they lived 100 miles away from you. Whether you are traveling or renting space, it all comes with a price.

Establishing a Business Entity - Independent Personal Trainer

To preface this section, talk to a business lawyer

and a certified public accountant on what fits your business model and long term plans. I am not a qualified legal consultant nor do I have enough insight for you to see the entire value of forming a limited liability corporation. Nonetheless, I will share with you why I chose to form an LLC to protect my personal assets and establish a legitimate organization.

Look into forming a limited liability corporation if you are going to be an independent personal trainer. When you are working as an employee at a gym, your employers may have established the company as a business entity (i.e. LLC, Corporation, etc.). Another great part of being an employee is that you are, in most instances, protected from liabilities under the company structure.

As an LLC, you're generating profit through the services you provide your clients. You would pay yourself, as an employee, a certain percentage of profits for services rendered. That paycheck is your money and therefore, part of your personal assets. The rest of profits are kept in your business for general business expenses, such as taxes, supplies, travel reimbursement and marketing. If a customer files a lawsuit against your company, then your personal assets are usually protected. There are exceptions to this rule and can be covered by a qualified business lawyer.

And of course, you will want a business account at your preferred banking institution. Having a business bank account should be part of your business model. If you are making money as a company, but depositing it into your personal account, once again, you are not functioning like an actual business. Could you imagine a fast food employee depositing the restaurants earnings into their personal bank account, then paying himself as he saw fit? This is not logical and would not be a good way to conduct your business. All earnings should go into a business bank account, and then you collect pay according to your business model. Track all payments with hours worked and your pay rate. When it comes time to file your taxes, everything will be in proper order for you certified public accountant to handle with ease.

Personal Training to Group Training

Personal training has evolved a lot in the last decade I've been involved. The traditional sense of personal training used to mean a fitness professional and client working one-on-one. That is, one personal trainer works with one client. This is, by far, my favorite type of training. I like to have that one-on-one connection with my clients. I learned more about that person, gained more insight on what motivated him and his perspective. And, the client received my undivided attention in the one-on-one session.

A drastic shift happened around late-2008 as the American economy took a nosedive. The customers and clients had less discretionary expenses, so they looked into cheaper alternatives to their health and fitness needs. As a personal trainer, I had to adjust to the demand of the market. I began working with more couples, small groups of friends and people looking for a large group to divide the training cost. With my attention divided I offered a price break for each client within that session.

Then, what revolutionized the business was the boot camp model. It was a group format with high-intensity interval training with multiple participants. Initially, I was steadfast against this format because I believed it devalued personal training. However, other trainers were becoming successful with this new concept. These boot camp trainers were getting larger paychecks and growing a raving fan base. Clients loved their sessions and would give referrals—not just for the group training, but for one-on-one training as well. My resolve broke and I looked into group training as an alternative to fill empty time slots and provide an additional revenue stream.

Consider this cost model:
1) Personal training session rate - $50 total profit
2) Couple training session rate - $40 per person = $80 total profit
3) Group training session rate - $20 per person = $60 - $240 total profit

(based on a 3-12 client threshold)

I realized I could affect more people in less time through group training. So, I changed my approach to accommodate larger groups. In the gym, I advertised group sessions and quickly filled my free time. Potential clients, who had previously passed on my services due to cost, jumped at the opportunity. Gym members who were hesitant before in personal training were eager to sign up for these groups.

And the greatest part was I had clients who transitioned from group training to personal training. Conversely, some personal training clients shifted to group training when they couldn't afford one-on-one training or they just needed maintenance workouts. The clients enjoyed the camaraderie in the group sessions and felt the sessions went quicker with more people involved.

Building Your Clientele

Building your clientele is different from being an employee at a gym to being an independent personal trainer. As I mentioned, in a gym you have members that you can use for finding clients. As an independent personal trainer, it's going to take more work in building your client list.

Referrals, or suggestions of people who may want to work with you, are one of the best ways of developing your business. Who do you know that would be interested in your personal training services? You must communicate with people what you do and ask around on who would be interested in your services. Get involved with social media and go to networking group meetings. You can probably find these on an online search of your area or through your local Chamber of Commerce. Some Chambers of Commerce offer two to three free visits which can help you establish contact with other people in your neighborhood. Though membership in your local Chamber of Commerce is not cheap, if you maximize the most out of this networking opportunity, then you will see your business explode.

Establishing a Community Presence

Regardless of your role, employee or business owner, establishing a community presence should be part of any successful business model. Get out and meet people in your community. There's no sign hanging above your head that reads "Personal Trainer." You need to network with other business associates, peers and people in your neighborhood. You can even set up some decent meet-up groups through websites and apps like MeetUp.com, Craigslist or other websites. For instance, you could organize or participate in groups interested in fitness, nutrition or healthy lifestyles.

The purpose of networking is to build

relationships and develop a rapport with people. There is a good chance that someone, who is impressed with your professionalism, will refer clients to you. So, don't badger people to invest in your personal training sessions—no one likes a pushy salesman.

Become involved in charity events, non-profit organizations or fundraisers that align with your personal and professional values. As a personal trainer, whether an employee or an independent trainer, you could donate to a raffle or a silent auction for charity. That's an excellent way to give back to the community and you will feel a sense of pride from helping those in need.

The advantage of helping others is that you get more exposure and attract more clients. For example, if you give personal training sessions, the person awarded the sessions may like your services enough to buy more from you. If you make a good impression, they are going to share with other people that they know, "I picked up these sessions at a silent auction and it was awesome. You will love this personal trainer. Go check him out!"

You are only limited by your imagination in how you interact with your community. I knew a trainer that would set up a table at a park and had cold beverages to hydrate the runners passing by. He would greet the runners and hand them a cold drink. This kind gesture opened an opportunity to build relationships with fitness-minded people who wanted to get a trainer. Most people would go about their day whereas others would stop and talk with him. After he repeatedly set up his booth, people began to recognize him and were more receptive to getting to know him. If you were to adopt this type of marketing, be sure you get permission from your local parks and recreation department.

Client Retention

Part of growing and maintaining your business is not only about acquiring clients but in keeping them. Client retention relies on how you conduct yourself and how you interact with your clientele. Every session needs to be unique and strictly focused on your client. You have to make the appointment about them.

Way Too Personal

A common mistake I made was in getting too familiar with my clients—meaning I shared a little too much of my personal affairs. Sharing my personal life took the focus away from my client and cheapened their time with me. They paid to hear about my expertise, not my personal life. Also, when you become buddies with your client, you become less of an authority on fitness and more of a pal who knows about fitness. Learn to separate your personal life from your working life. It's okay to share a particular life experience to clarify a point. But, if you are only talking about your love life or favorite movies, then you have shared too much.

Though you are a personal trainer, remember, your client invests in your personal training, not your personal life. If a client asks you about your personal life, answer briefly, and then focus on the session. If you have less than 30 to 60 minutes of working with your client, then that's a brief time within their day. Depending on the number of times per week or per month you see your client, that is less than one hour out of 168 within a week or about 5,040 within a month.

You would be completely remiss if you took the focus away from your client. There's never a lack of things to talk relevant to your client's goals within a half-hour to an hour time slot. Discuss their outside activities, their nutrition or their progress. Additionally, you can:
1. Instruct and correct exercise form
2. Count repetitions
3. Discuss exercise programming
4. Offer support
5. Encourage them
6. Suggest groups they can get involved in
7. Talk about any other information pertinent to their wants and needs.
8. It never hurts to repeat what you say to your clients.

Client retention depends on how you conduct yourself and how you maintain order within the session. Make the appointment the most important and fun time in your client's day. After all, you have little time to influence your client. Make your workout together a fantastic experience and they will want to come back for more.

If you keep clients on track and they meet their goals, then you increase the likelihood of them continuing to invest in you. Remember to always look ahead and know their next objective. Try to revisit their plans throughout your sessions together. That way they aren't surprised when it's time to buy sessions in advance.

Client Retention Strategies & Advance Payment

Set your client's goals and expectations. Discuss how long it takes to achieve their goals and remind them about purchasing options. Let your client know your willingness to commit to a long-term plan to help them achieve their goals, but this requires an upfront investment. Through advanced purchasing, you could lay out a game plan for that period of time and adjust along the way to fit their needs.

Cancellation Policy

Also, establish a cancelation policy for all client agreements, and make sure that it can legally hold up in the event of a dispute. Many reasons prevent clients from making it to an appointment. Some excuses are valid and deserve a bit of compassion and understanding. However, other reasons are irrational and may represent a lack of respect for your time. But, in either situation, you must treat the situation with tact and professionalism. You have to decide if you charge your client for a missed session or not. In some instances, I would reschedule if time allowed. Other times, I would allow one absence, but remind the client of the cancelation policy. After all, if a client fills a time slot and doesn't show up, then they forfeit time you could otherwise fill with other clients.

A cancelation can be even more detrimental to an independent personal trainer. You can be on your way to a client's house or another location when you get a cancelation. That may waste valuable time and money. You're the one that's going to be inconvenienced.

If you charge a client for a missed session, be sure to tactfully inform them. Much like a missed doctor's appointment, the doctor charges the patient if he does not cancel within 24 hours of the session. Establish what your cancelation policy is and stick to it. Stay consistent with the cancelation policy regardless of the relationships you build—long-term or short-term. All clients should be treated equally.

Chapter Four - Personal Training Practice

Advertising & Marketing Your Business

If you want more clients, then you have to market or advertise your services. If you are an employee of a gym, you may have a sales team responsible for getting gym members. In turn, you can market directly to an audience in the comforts of your workplace.

I knew a trainer who would distribute flyers throughout nearby apartment complexes or on car windshields in his downtime (with permission). Helping the sales force brought in additional gym patrons. In turn, he had a larger pool of potential clients.

In my downtime at the gym, I kept busy by cleaning up equipment, making the gym tidy and interacting with people. I always made a point to stay active when I was in the gym. If a gym member were to see me sitting for too long, then their perception is that I probably don't have any clients. Worse yet, the perception is that I'm lazy if I'm sitting around. Remember, if you're at a desk for more than a half-hour to an hour, then that's a half-hour or an hour of a person's workout that they're watching you doing nothing. If you have to work at a desk, try to do it out of sight. It is better you're not seen than to be seen doing nothing.

As an independent trainer, you may have to look into advertising options. I'm fortunate that I developed enough of a reputation through word of mouth. When I became an independent personal trainer, I had an audience and plenty of referrals that advertising wasn't necessary. So, I made a rather successful living working part-time.

Consider using newspaper ads or flyers for advertising. Before you start posting flyers all over the place, make sure it's according to community codes and law. Get permission ahead of time for posting on private properties (i.e. apartments, condos, etc.). Some communities have a zero tolerance policy for solicitation, so tread with care.

Depending on your certifying organization, you may be able to post ads or a profile for free on their web directory. Some websites specialize in advertising your services including, Idea Fit, Groupon, Living Social, and more. You will always get what you pay for, so paying for more exposure may be necessary. Otherwise, you take your chances of being lost in hundreds of other products and fitness-related ads.

Building Leads

Building leads, or potential customers, is vital to the growth of your business. If you discover through a conversation with Tom that he is trying to lose weight but hasn't been working out for quite some time, then there is a good chance you may have a solution for him. Make sure you take note of that or begin a spreadsheet on your computer of your lead.

I used to have a notebook I used to keep tabs on the interaction, the relevant topic, and the person. This tracked my leads, so that way I knew how to follow up with people. Make connections with everyone and most importantly, remember their name. People love to hear their name. Don't forget to identify that person by his name every time you see him. Say, "Hey, Tom! How are your workouts going?"

Be sincere in your engagement. You shouldn't just be fishing for the next client, but remember this person is a potential client. When you have an open time slot or a cancelation, you can stay busy by filling that time with a potential client. You could say, "Hey Tom, I know you've been working your tail off and I had a cancelation. I'd rather work with somebody than nobody at all. It would be a big favor to me if you wouldn't mind jumping in for a session with me."

Then, you would be working with someone as opposed to doing nothing during that time. You're providing a good service, developing rapport, and also giving a test drive of your services. Additionally, other people in the gym see how well you work rather than how good you do nothing.

It's different as an independent trainer, especially if you run a mobile service. If you have a cancelation while en route to your client's house, then you could search your leads to find someone to fill the appointment. Call around to find out who is available and willing to work with you. Other clients may be eager to fill the empty time, so never overlook bringing additional value to your loyal customers. You can do any number of things and the only limit is your imagination and willingness to try something new.

Honest Feedback to Improve Quality

Honest feedback is what helps you improve your services and attentiveness to detail. I would briefly have my clients reflect on their session, post-workout. I ask questions, such as:

1) What are your honest feelings about this session?
2) How well do you feel it went?
3) What did you like best about the session?
4) On a scale of 0 to 10—0 being the worst session ever and 10 being the best thing you've ever experienced—where was today's workout on that scale?

Listen carefully to their answers and evaluate each from a third person perspective. Avoid getting caught up in taking their responses personally, regardless of how they like or dislike the day's routine. Absolutely do not interrupt them or become defensive. Follow up with some additional questions, such as:

1) What would make the session a (higher rating)? - Based on their answer, ask what would make it 1 point greater than their answer. If it was a 10, then you may have a winner of a workout.
2) What did you like best about the workout?
3) What would make the workout a (lower rating)? - Based on their answer, ask what would make it 2-3 points less than their answer. If it was a 1, then you may want to reevaluate your approach to training this person and working on building better rapport.
4) What did you like least about the workout?

Think of how you can constructively use that information and make your future sessions better for that client. Bear in mind, not all answers represent all clients' feeling, but what you do with the information will improve you as a trainer. Be responsive not only to your client's needs but their wants. Then you are providing stellar service. And, avoid making self-deprecating comments in light of the negative feedback. It minimizes your client's feedback and leaves them feeling less valued for their candid opinions.

Asking for Referrals & Testimonials

As you meet client expectations, you can easily segue into tactfully asking for referrals or testimonials. Referrals, or recommendations to use your services, are what keep your business afloat without any overhead cost on marketing or advertising. When a customer is happy with your services, then he is apt to share. And, to make the process even easier for your clients, you can have them tell who would be most interested in your services. For instance, you could say, "Tom, I know you've enjoyed our sessions and wondered - do you know anyone who would be interested in my training?"

Make it brief and avoid hounding your clients for referrals. This approach is not a sales tactic to bring you tons of revenue. It should be a casual while respecting your client's space and time to decide. If they know of someone, then ask if you could arrange a session with that person. Another easy way to get a referral is to have your client invite them to a buddy session. Have the referral try your services while being with your client.

Usually during workouts, your client may discuss his interactions with friends or family. You'll often hear a recurring person maybe a wife, friend or co-worker. In getting to know your client, you may become aware of their peers and sense who would be most interested in joining a session. You can always say, "Hey, next week, if you'd like to, I can make a buddy session for you both. I won't charge you anything for that person for this one time. Bring him in."

That's going to be up to you and your comfort level. And if you're working for an employer, get permission from your direct supervisor. As an independent trainer, it's up to you if you are willing to try this approach to grow your business. It seems counter-intuitive to what I advised before in that you shouldn't devalue your service. But, this is an easier and cheaper method as opposed to paying for advertisements and marketing.

When you first build your business, be prepared to offer free sessions often. Don't allow anyone to abuse this service. For instance, your client, Tom, may bring along his close friend, Bob, for a free session. Bob has a great workout and you hit it off with him. You could say after the appointment, "I would love to work with you again, is there any chance I could work with you one-on-one?"

Though you may have given your best efforts, Bob declines. Then, ask Bob for permission to keep in contact and you can always keep him in your leads list.

If you suggest to your client, Tom, to bring a friend along again, be sure that you explicitly state that a free session is only good once per person. You are devaluing your service if people are getting more than one free session. People love most anything free and complimentary personal training sessions are rarely turned down when you are an in-demand trainer. Opt for one sample per person.

Another way to get more work is through testimonials from your existing clientele. If someone is happy with your service and expresses it on a regular basis, then ask for a simple testimonial. Generate your own testimonial questionnaire for your client to fill in. The information should collect the following:

1) A client picture or before & after photos, if applicable. Be sure to have a client photo release document signed before producing the testimonial.
2) What was life before your personal training sessions?
3) What did your client find when he came to you?
4) What did your client accomplish with you?
5) What does your client plan on doing next? And, will it be in your services? If not, then what has your client learned from you to do confidently on their own?
6) Would your client recommend you to other people?

Free Group Training Classes for Multiple Leads

Set up free group training classes as a way to draw in additional leads and clients. When you have downtime, you can always set up free classes. Try to set it up one to four weeks in advance so you can advertise and spread the news through word of mouth. Free classes can be super easy. Use an email list to send out notifications or a campaign informing them of your free group training class. Additionally, people love incentives, so offer a door prize to encourage early arrival. This early bird incentive keeps your class flowing on time and decreases distractions from late arrivals. A simple email would read like this:

> *My schedule is available on Monday from 3:30 p.m. to 4:30 p.m., so I'm going to host a free yoga class at the clubhouse. Please let me know whether or not you'll make it. The first five people to arrive will receive a free workout towel.*
>
> *Sincerely,*
> *Dale*

Don't let the class begin without having all

attendees sign in. Have a form for your attendees to fill out their names, their numbers, and their email addresses. Remember that the free class is not only providing an excellent service; you are looking for potential leads. Also, for best business practice, I recommend having attendees sign a liability waiver. When your class finishes, get them pumped up and excited. Your attendees are going to be flying on a workout high and if you can get them leaving your class energized and bustling about the class, other people will be curious about joining your future sessions.

Much like a one-on-one training session, have the group give feedback at the end of the session. Ask something like, "Let's see a show of hands. Who would like to come to future classes like this?" If they put their hands up, that's great! You may want to continue doing a group training class with these people, especially if they develop camaraderie as a group.

After group training sessions, people gather together in small groups and talk for a bit. Those are the people you could possibly put into small group sessions. Or, you can get them to try out a one-on-one session.

Remember, limit the number of free sessions with people. Beyond a free group training session, I offer only one free personal training session per person. If the group wishes to do another session together, then develop a training package to accommodate the group. Avoid continually offering free classes to the same group of people.

Remember to hang on to those leads, because your leads list helps fill your schedule. Follow up with your leads and don't be afraid to call them. "Hey, how are you doing?"

Establish a purpose for your call. "Hey, there's a reason why I'm calling you, Tom." Then share with them what you're calling them for—whether you have an empty time slot or a free group training session. Now, of course, don't hassle them or try to sell personal training sessions.

Before making any phone call, be sure that your lead is comfortable with you calling. You aren't a telemarketer and you shouldn't be cold calling or contacting someone you don't have a relationship with.

Getting to Know Your Client

A personal training career requires making a connection with each client so that you provide the best service according to their wants and needs. If you don't know your clients or why they want your services, then your business will fail. If you have only one client, but you know them real well, then you are on track to running a successful business.

In the first session with your client, find out his purpose or reason for why he wants to use your services. Some questions to ask your client are:

1) What do you want to accomplish?
2) Why are deciding to make a change?
3) Why is this your priority now?
4) Why are you coming to me instead of trying it on your own?
5) What are your long term goals?

As an expert in your field, help your client set realistic and measurable goals. If you cannot measure or quantify an outcome, then how will you know when you have arrived at your destination? Can you actually measure feeling better, toning up or losing weight? Get to the root cause of why your client wants to feel better. Nobody wants to fail, but if your client doesn't set realistic and measurable goals, then they're increasing the likelihood of disappointment and failure.

It can be a complicated process to flush out answers, but remember that you aren't there to make your client feel uncomfortable, awkward or embarrassed. You aren't a psychotherapist and shouldn't dish out advice on body image issues, or suggest how to cope with deep-seeded issues. You merely provide sound advice on what you know best—health and fitness. If at first you don't discover exactly what your client is shooting for, in due time, you will begin to gain a better understanding of why your client is there and how you can best help them.

Set expectations when it comes to measurable

goals. If you determine that losing ten pounds can be done over the course of ten weeks, then set that expectation. Set the timeline with a finish date for the ten-pound weight loss. You can set goals according to your education and experience. Evaluate goals and expectations along the way, making sure your client is on track to meeting his goal.

"I'm excited about you losing ten pounds. How are things going?" They'll express to you how things are going.

"How have your independent workouts been?"

"Oh, my workouts have been fantastic."

"Awesome! Were you able to get that cardio workout in?"

"Oh, I wasn't able to make it."

"Well, that's all right. We're still gonna make that ten pounds." Adjust the expectations a bit according to the client update.

Continue to mention your client's goals, how he will fulfill them and applaud any progress he has made. Your client should be excited when he sees you and cannot wait to get back with you in the next session.

Preparing for Appointments

Always arrive on time for every session. You're on time if you're five minutes early. You're late if you show up on time. And if you show up five minutes late, then you need to make it up to your client. This is no hard and fast rule you have to adhere to every time. Should you ever be late for an appointment, finish at the scheduled time and don't charge for the session. And, avoid making every appointment late after the first one. Better that one appointment is late rather than all of them.

Regardless, you should always be on time and ready for your appointments. Time is invaluable, not only for you as a personal trainer, but also for your client. They invest both their money and their time. The greatest disservice and disrespect is to throw away or cheapen a person's time.

In my business model, I had two types of sessions—half-hour and hour sessions. This is not to say I trained my client for 30 minutes or 60 minutes straight. I finish up 27 minutes into a half hour session and 55 minutes into an hour session. The final minutes of a session is for confirming information with the current client, filing notes and preparing for the next appointment. As an example, if one session is at 6:00 p.m., then I prepare for it at 5:58 p.m. When a half-hour appointment is set for 5:30 p.m., I'm wrapping up the session by 5:57 p.m. Additionally, if an hour appointment is set for

5:00 p.m., then I stop at 5:55 p.m. The reason you need more time after an hour session is to file more information compiled from the longer session.

Inform your first-time clients how a session is timed. People are more appreciative when you are upfront about how you do business.

Know how you scheduled your day, and then have everything set up in advance. If your workday is from 6:00 a.m. to 2:00 p.m., then you should have all programs organized and laid out so you are ready for each one. You should be able to pull a client file out, familiarize yourself with their unique conditions and goals and have the entire session planned out. By having all plans laid out for the day, you can transition from one appointment to the other with little stress.

The first thing you should always do for every appointment is to inform your client of what to expect in the session. When you set expectations up front, you almost assure victory for everyone. Then, you both are on the same page and can work cohesively. Your explanation should be no more than a thirty-second overview of the workout.

When you inform your client of the game plan, you flush out any potential issues that may inhibit the workout. Your client can tell you about excessive soreness, an injury or even where his mindset is before the session. At this point, you push forward according to plan or make some last minute changes according to what you have learned about your client.

Be ready and have a backup plan for unexpected news or problems. New fitness professional may find some difficulty having a backup plan or improvising. Be open and honest with your client and tell them your revised plan.

My first year in the business, I was a nervous wreck when I had to change plans. If this happens to you, then, take a deep breath first. Relax and remember that they know you're not super human. Then express to them, "Look if you bear with me, I'm still going to give you a great session today. Since we're going to have to modify things, it's going to probably be at a more deliberate pace than usual. Do you mind?" Most clients will understand or in some instances, reschedule so that you can adequately plan for the sudden change. In this case, do not charge a client for a rescheduled appointment.

The Client's First Appointment

When you schedule your client's first appointment, be sure to confirm 24-48 hours in advance of the session. When you call to confirm your appointment, expect to briefly answer any questions your client has and defuse any objections or reservations. Tell your client what to expect in the first appointment, what to bring and where to meet. Beyond that, save all of your discussion time to the appointment where you can comfortably ask him person-to-person what his goals and expectations are in your services.

Wait at the meetup location a few minutes before the start of the session. Greet your client in an uplifting, energetic way with a simple handshake. Introduce yourself and ask what your client prefers to be called. A simple step like this seems common sense; however, I have had some unfortunate experiences based on how I mispronounced names and even called people by the wrong name. Here's a best practice—repeat their name three times within the first five minutes of meeting them. You shouldn't have much trouble remembering their name for the rest of the session and future appointments.

Your first experience with anyone should be getting to know them. Don't take a person right into exercises without first learning about them. This protects their health and your career. While you learn a bit more about their wishes, you should learn about any pre-existing conditions and precautions. They may not have any health conditions, but that doesn't necessarily mean they are prepared for a vigorous routine. Some people aren't physically equipped for a workout and require careful exercise selection.

First, fill out pertinent information, including:
1) Basic client information - name, contact information
2) Liability waiver and/or informed

consent

3) PAR-Q - physical activity readiness questionnaire

4) Doctor release forms - when a client has pre-existing conditions that you are not able to address, be sure that you refer out or get a doctor's release. Do not work with a client with special needs without getting this important document completed.

5) Photo release - if a client refuses, do not press the issue. Some people have body image issues and would rather not get pictures. Or they may be willing to get pictures on their own.

6) Goal planning sheet

Most gyms provide these forms for their training staff. If you're an independent trainer, most certification programs come with necessary forms and templates for you to use.

After they have filled out their personal info, go through the information with them to clarify answers and ask additional questions. Next, have your client read through the liability waiver/informed consent. These forms inform your client of the inherent risks in working out. Typically, those two items come in one form, but some companies keep them entirely separate. Confirm with your certifying organization or your liability insurance for what is the best practice for your type of personal training.

In the rare instances of incident, injury or fatality, these forms are your safety net, so never take them lightly nor pass them off as unessential. Most personal training liability insurance plans would not cover the expenses of litigation if the trainer did not have the liability waiver completed before the session. If somebody refuses to sign it, then stop the session until the client is comfortable with signing this form. In those instances, he needs to be fully informed about what he is signing and why he is signing it.

After all, the completed forms are in the best interest of you, your business, and that person's health. The truth is there are going to be risks in every workout. Assure your client it is not your intention to harm them and you will make every precaution necessary for a safe workout.

The next thing is to identify any medical conditions or diagnoses that require special attention or modifications in the workout. Some health conditions include:
    1) High blood pressure
    2) Diabetes
    3) Asthma
    4) Any condition requiring medication

Before the first workout, have your client with medical conditions obtain a doctor's consent. This form is another item you can get from your certifying organization. Your client's primary care physician needs to know his patient is working with you and the type of training regimen you plan to use. Then the doctor can make recommendations and any contraindications according to your client's needs.

Instruct and train according to the best interests of your client. So, inform your client your need for a doctor's consent so you provide the safest, most effective programming. If your client has any reservations, then you can offer to reach out to his doctor. This is as simple as finding out the doctor's name, address and phone number. Contact the doctor's office and explain the situation and what you are looking for to provide your client a safe routine. The few occasions I had to do this, the doctor's office was always willing to work with me. The rare occasions that I didn't have the doctor's consent before a session, I would reschedule the session a week or so away until I had the completed form.

Goal Setting on the First Appointment

There needs to be a purpose—a reason why your client is choosing to use your services. Whether they are doing marathons or they're looking to lose thirty pounds—there should be a desired outcome for your client. With your client, set goals that have a measurable and time-specific outcome. Come to an agreement with your client and offer options rather than force them to see your point of view. You may be the expert, but if they don't entirely agree with you, then they may not follow any of your recommendations. Offer sound advice both of you agree to. This is where your education will come into play and you should share evidence of why your guidance is sound and logical. And, express this information in a friendly, non-confrontational way. You want to inform your client, not alienate them.

Find out the importance of a goal. Ask how life would be better or improved by completing the goal. Be sure to track all the information shared and don't rely on your memory alone. Whether you write it down or put it on your mobile device, this information is helpful in developing the best exercise program. Eventually, you'll review your notes with your client.

After you agree on the goals, take measurements using a scale, tape measure, body fat monitor and a camera. Largely dependent on their goals, you may not need these tools. If someone is training for a marathon, then you will need tests relevant to their outcome. An example of a basic test would be a one-mile run for someone training for long-distance running. Your certifying organization determines what tests or measurements are necessary to your client's goals.

The first day should be when you first measure so that you have a baseline. Then, set a follow-up date at thirty, sixty and ninety days out to re-evaluate progress.

Also, get a good picture of your client. Inform your client, it is merely for their chart and you will only use the image with their permission. One of the great ways to keep your files organized is having a photo of your client. This is also an excellent way for your client to look back at the before image after getting results.

Always confirm the next appointment with your client before the session is over. I can't tell you how much heartache I had by not confirming appointments and someone wouldn't show and they said, "You never told me." Even though they booked the session, you're still at a loss. Sure you can charge them if you have a cancelation policy. But, you want to work with your clients to get results. So, it never hurts to overcommunicate.

Setting Your Schedule

The more successful I became, the more my time filled up. Eventually, I had to book beyond my regular hours. Before long, my days were stretched to 12-hour days with scattered half-hour breaks throughout the day. It was hard to sustain that type of schedule because I sacrificed my time for the betterment of others. Sure, I made significant money, but I never enjoyed the spoils of my hard work.

Set a realistic schedule and stick to it.

If you went to a restaurant at 9:05 p.m. and it closes at 9:00 p.m., how likely are they going to stay open to accommodate you? In this instance, you would have to come back the next day if you want to eat there. This circumstance applies to your business as well. It is a service-based industry where you need to set and honor scheduled hours. Don't compromise your time because you're looking to get as many clients as you can. If you develop a strong enough presence and brand, then people will wait for an available opening.

Of course, I burned out because I worked long days with no rest. When I discussed the issue with my manager, she gave me advice that serves me well to this day—set your schedule and stick to it.

You can set up a wait list or add the potential clients to your leads list. Follow up with your potential clients while they wait for your services. See what you can provide and help them with in the meantime. An encouraging word can go a long way and updates give them a sense of importance in your business.

Chapter Five - Do's & Don'ts

This book was largely developed from my years of fielding questions from hopeful personal trainers. Some people I spoke to about personal training had some experience and others were entertaining a personal training career. Outside of some of the fundamentals I previously covered, there are a few topics I feel need to be covered. However, I couldn't categorize these miscellaneous items under anything other than do's and don'ts.

Honestly & Openly Communicate with Your Clients

Always openly express any scheduling conflicts or any leave of absence with your clientele. Be straightforward and honest with your clients even if you feel awkward or fear losing business.

If you have to leave town for awhile, then inform your clients ahead so they can make plans. Offer a substitute trainer for the meantime, and confirm your clients are comfortable with a substitution. Communicate up front with your clients.

A personal trainer planned on an extended vacation and needed my assistance in training her clientele during her absence. She did a great job introducing me to her clients and had me shadow a few sessions. Additionally, I ran a couple to make sure I'd meet their approval. But, when it came time for her absence, she left on her trip with not so much a word to her clients of my prolonged substitution. After quite a few sessions, the clients suspected what was going on and asked me. This left me in an awkward position having to explain to her clientele what actually happened.

Fortunately, her clients liked me and our sessions together were wonderful. Even if you think you will lose clients when you leave for an extended period of time, tell them the truth. Restaurants close for business when they have to be remodeled or are low-staffed. Television shows go on a hiatus between seasons. And, personal trainers need a vacation once in awhile. Rather than worry about losing business, respect your customers and inform them of an interruption in service. Offer to set up a substitution, and then book a follow-up appointment for after your return.

How to Carry Yourself in a Session

How you carry yourself makes all the difference in your customer's perception of you. There's a definite difference between being professional and unprofessional. Here are a few suggestions on how to conduct yourself as a fitness professional.

LEANING
Don't lean against equipment, the wall or anything else. You project an uncaring attitude when you prop yourself up. Or, worse yet, you

give the impression that you're too lazy to stand up. Now, I'm not telling you to stand around like you have a stick up your ass, but you do have to carry yourself with relaxed poise.

HOVERING
Don't hover over your clients. If they're doing floor exercises, kneel down and remove most of the separation between you and your client. Maintain a close distance while respecting their personal space. If you need to spot a client on an exercise, then you may have to come in close. Inform first-time clients your intentions when you come into their personal space.

Remember, people are watching. If you are seen hovering over your clients with your arms crossed, then you may be perceived as a tough drill sergeant out to break all of his recruits.

PHONE ETIQUETTE
Put your phone away during a session. If you have your phone in your hand—looking through texts or making a call—you will be perceived as being disinterested in your clients. Playing with your phone during your session is unprofessional. I would be horrified if I was at a restaurant and in the middle of taking an order, my server would answer his phone and start talking. I would certainly leave the establishment and discourage anyone from ever going there.

Put your phone on silent. When you use it for business, tell your clientele. But, remember that people are watching and other people don't know that you're not texting or playing around with apps. Be appropriate with how you are taking notes. Using a tablet or an iPad removes some of the ambiguity so people have less doubt about what you are doing. Use mobile technology with discretion.

You're Always on Stage - People Are Watching

Perception is always a subjective reality. If every weekday, a gym patron walks on a treadmill for a half hour and they see you sitting at a desk every time, then their perception is that you don't work. They don't know you're answering emails or planning programs for the next three months. What they see is a worker, who may or may not be a trainer, who sits a lot and spends all his time on the computer. Keep your sitting time limited from five to ten minutes. Do a little work, and then go talk to people and move around a bit. Do any significant amount of work out of sight.

One day, as I was racking up weights, a coworker and I happened to look over at this trainer. This gentleman would spend a lot of time behind a desk working on his administrative tasks (i.e. emails, programs, etc.) and this particular day was no exception. A long line of cardio equipment on the second-floor loft overlooked the line of desks at the front of the gym. Picture windows were directly behind the desks with an open view to the parking lot.

As we tidied the dumbbell rack, we happened to look over to see this trainer knuckle-deep in his nose. No mistake about it, he was definitely working, but not in the traditional sense. Cleaning out your nose should be kept in discrete locations.

If you are doing cartwheels, screaming at people, throwing equipment, then no one will want to work with you. Unless you're a drill sergeant, you should never be shouting. Nobody outside of your training session understands this unprofessional behavior.

Avoid talking outside of your session. You will have various distractions threatening to interrupt your session. Some people will become familiar with you and want to carry a conversation.

Merely state, "Hey, I'll catch up with you later."

People should respect that you are working with your client and let you continue your job. Your clients are investing in you and your time so you should keep them the center of your attention.

Clean Up After Yourself

Clean up during and after your sessions. Often, I have clients clean up or do it myself during workouts. If I need them to continue an exercise that is safe without my assistance, I will clean up then. Cleanliness is about safety for everyone.

Additionally, if you have three to five minutes free time between your sessions—that should be clean up time. Pick up exercise mats, put away steppers, and hang up jump ropes. Regardless of whose mess it is, clutter is a hazard. Set a good example and clean up regularly.

Inspect the Equipment You Use

Always inspect the equipment you use in training sessions. You could do this at the start of your day, before a session, during clean up or throughout your session. Even though you've seen some equipment many times, check it out anyway. Never use beat up, worn out, cracked or frayed equipment. When in doubt, throw it out, or put an "Out of Order" sign on it. You have a responsibility as a personal trainer to know when something is not safe for anyone. If you personally don't want to use it, then chances are other people shouldn't use it either.

Mobile fitness trainers should definitely know what their equipment looks like and the condition it's in. If it starts to fray, to break or seem questionable, toss it out. Broken equipment becomes a liability, especially if you're aware of it.

Body Image Issues

Use discretion with clients who have body image issues. Some people are self-conscious enough that they don't like to have measurements taken, pictures snapped or to be placed in front of a group of people in their workouts. Try to empathize, or see where they are in their struggle, and do your best to accommodate them.

I had some clients that broke down crying because they didn't want to step on a scale or to be in front of a mirror. It's a significant victory for a person to overcome their fears and work with you. Focus on the things you can do within your sessions rather than on the things you can't. Avoid minimizing any fears and do the best you can with what they are comfortable doing.

Don't make it a battle convincing them do what you want. Otherwise, you're making the training session about you rather than about them. Any session spent arguing or forcing your point of view on a client is time wasted, because no one likes being wrong. And, next, if it was a struggle for them to show up for the appointment, then it will be that much harder knowing that you are out to prove them wrong the next time they see you.

Be aware of where your client is and the direction she is performing her movements at all times. Certain exercises can offer compromising views of private areas. You don't want to showcase all their glory to everyone in the gym. Sometimes you can position yourself in a way to block prying eyes—if not to protect your client, then to avoid indirectly making other self-conscious people more aware of their own body image issues.

Mindfully Choose Exercise Space & Share

Be considerate of other people outside of your session and share the space when you train large groups. Whether it's in a park or a gym, you will take up a lot of room with a group of twelve or more people. I knew a trainer that was incredibly successful and had a few groups of a dozen people each. Every time he moved his group to an area, he monopolized the entire area and inadvertently pushed every other person out of the way. Be mindful and respect everybody's space.

Conclusion

When I started in the personal training business, I had some of the greatest mentors in the business and awesome peers—all of them were great fitness professionals. I learned and grew because of them and wouldn't have been half as successful if it weren't for their teamwork and willingness to help me.

This book was a compilation of all I learned from the trainers, managers and fitness professionals I worked with over the past decade in this business. It's my hope that you get as much info from this book as you can so you can realize your breakthroughs quicker than I did. And, on your path to becoming a successful personal trainer, you, too, will learn your own lessons that may not even be listed in this book. Remember to keep learning, growing, developing and working at becoming extraordinary in this field by helping others achieve their definition of greatness.

It's one thing to learn from someone who is experienced and has had success in this line of work. But it's essential that you actually apply what you have learned. You, too, may have a successful career if you take the right steps. So, get out there, don't be afraid, and give it your best. After all, you can make a change in this world when you become a Consummate Fitness Professional.

About The Author

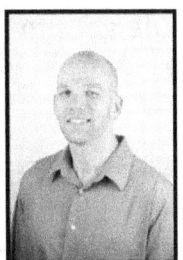

My name is Dale Lewis Roberts and I'm a former American Council on Exercise Personal Trainer, Certified, with an ACE Specialty Certification in Senior Fitness. Since beginning my personal training career in 2006, I earned numerous certifications in personal training, yoga, nutritional coaching, among others. I have worked with hundreds of clients with a variety of health & fitness goals.

While my greatest passions are health & fitness, writing and reading, I also love to spend time traveling with my wife, watching pro wrestling and playing guitar. I currently reside in Phoenix, Arizona, with my wife, Kelli, and our rescue cat, Izzie.

Special Thanks

The highest gratitude goes to my wife, Kelli; and my best buddies, Harold Webb, and Russ Webster.

My old LFF buddies: Rob Emge, Mike Osgood, Bob Davis, Elizabeth Ellis English, Jon Mayle, Esteban Lutz and Kevin Maag for all of your contributions to my early growth and success as a trainer. Caitlin (Renner) Trainer, Natalie Barry, Jake Handschke, Jessica (Adams) Aun, Todd Cunningham, Heather Kiley.

My old clients: Kris K., Carol Langkamp, Kara & Scott Selby, Jeff Selby, Jenny Chafin, Angie Lowe, Geoff & Susie Delman, Laura Critzer, the ladies of Code Pink Boot Camp (July 2014 - October 2014), Yvette Graser.

My Facebook followers & friends: Ankit Garg, Susan Parks, Mark Perring, Keith Oliver, Pennie Dodson, Wild Bill, Matt Ryan, Jennifer Essinger, Amy Alt MacGuire.

This book is dedicated to my dad, Mike Roberts, and my mother, Kaye Cox. I have the two best parents a son could ever ask for. Both your hard work ethic rubbed off on me and has served me well for many years. I love you both with all my heart and any amount of success I get is a reflection of your parenting.

Get a free audiobook download of *The Consummate Fitness Professional* with a 30-day trial of Audible today!

Head over to:
US Region -
https://dalelroberts.com/fitpro
UK Region -
https://dalelroberts.com/fitproUK
FR Region -
https://dalelroberts.com/fitproFR
DE Region -
https://dalelroberts.com/fitproDE

References

[i] Merriam-Webster, Inc. (2015, May 5). Definition of demographic. Retrieved from http://www.merriam-webster.com/dictionary/demographic

[ii] Salary.com. (2015, May 9). Personal Trainer Salaries. Retrieved from http://www1.salary.com/Personal-Trainer-Salary.html

[iii] Merriam-Webster, Inc. (2015, May 21). Definition of credibility. Retrieved from http://www.merriam-webster.com/dictionary/credibility

[iv] Dictionary.com. (2015, May 10). Definition of liable. Retrieved from http://dictionary.reference.com/browse/liable?s=t

www.ingramcontent.com/pod-product-compliance
Lightning Source LLC
Chambersburg PA
CBHW070756290526
45795CB00002B/571